A Diagnostic Primer of Case Reports and Words of Wisdom

Dedicated to my 4 daughters----who are all nurses

BY

Paul W. Holtzman, M.D.

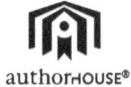

authorHOUSE®

AuthorHouse™
1663 Liberty Drive
Bloomington, IN 47403
www.authorhouse.com
Phone: 1-800-839-8640

First published by AuthorHouse 7/1/2009

ISBN: 978-1-4389-7722-5 (sc)

Printed in the United States of America
Bloomington, Indiana

This book is printed on acid-free paper.

Resume

Indiana University	1944	B.S. Medicine
Indiana University	1947	M.D.
Interneship	1947-48	Youngstown Ohio General Hospital
General Residency	1948-49	Bluffton Clinic, Bluffton, Indiana
Internal Medicine residency 1st yr	1949-50	Toledo Hospital, Toledo, Ohio
2nd and 3rd yr res Int Med	1950-52	Indianapolis General Hospital
Entered Private practice	1952--2004	Bloomington, Indiana

Contents

My idea to write this booklet came from my daughter. She was studying to become a nurse practioner and she really seemed to derive some benefit from reading simple case histories. Hence this attempt to portray the average day in a general practioners office.

THERE ARE SEVERAL BASIC RULES THAT APPLY TO ALL PRACTIONERS

1. If you don't know the answers—don't confabulate or lie—just say nothing. (The patient will mistakingly think you are a wise one who knows, but does't tell all) ONE CAN NEVER MAKE AN ASS OF HIMSELF BY KEEPING QUIET!

2. Always undress the patient if necessary-don't try to examine through a keyhole!

3. Patients may be shopping. They may have no intention of taking your medicine.. Therefore consider the patient "your patient" only when he or she is sitting directly in front of you across your desk.

4. Don't believe everything you are told. LISTEN AND EVALUATE.

Wife-------------he stuck me

Husband---------she's going out on me!

Grandmother----both are liars

Son--------------everything was okay til Grannie moved in our house.

5. X-ays and lab studies are just as good as the technicians who do the work.

6. DON'T try to save the patient money by not ordering what you deem necessary. Do not let cost effect dictate your choice of treatment.

7. Forget lawsuits—don't let lawyers dominate your decisions.

8. Do not let relatives dictate treatment. BUT do not underestimate the wisdom or experience of grandmothers.

9. Do not let the patient dictate treatment or medications prescribed.

10. FREQUENTLY THE HARDEST THING TO DO IS NOTHING!

11. DO NOT FORGET THAT MANY CONDITIONS ARE MADE WORSE BY THE IATROGENIC COMPONENT.

12. Do not think patients are medical geniuses or students of latin—tell them skin infection NOT DERMATITIS. Tell them inflammation of the muscle—NOT MYALGIA. Say headache—NOT CEPHALGIA. Say diahrrea—NOT GASTROENTERITIS.

13. Believe what patients say regarding allergy. If they say they are allergic to aspirin or penicillin—BELIEVE THEM.

14. If you don't gel with a patient—get an early divorce in the relationship. Treatment is based on mutual trust.

15. If the patient has a list of complaints—watch out!! One doesn't need a list to remember that they hit their finger with a hammer. IF THEY HAVE A LIST OR ARE CARRYING A PDR----WATCH OUT!!

16. Never, NEVER sit on the hospital bed of the patient. If you have ever been a patient and have the bed jostled when you are already

uncomfortable—you'll know what I mean. Besides, it is a dirty habit.

17. This is the most important—IF YOU LISTEN LONG ENOUGH, THE PATIENT WILL TELL YOU WHAT'S WRONG.

18. Always touch the patient. This may be a simple handshake or a pat on the back, but it will help establish rapport

When initiating conversation with a patient, don't say "what's wrong?" The reply will inevitable be "That's what I came here to find out". Begin with "What can I do for you?" or "How can I be of help to you?" Don't ever say 'how old are you?" for the answer will inevitably be " GUESS!" Don't ever ask the patient the color of their stools as they will say they never look. Instead, say "Are your stools black or clay colored?" In taking a history, don't be embarrassed to ask the questions you need to know---be humble with the patient. --- Take the "help me to help you approach"

At the appropriate time, ask the patient what he or she thinks is the problem—they usually know.

I'm sick and tired of hearing that 95% of the people who appear in the office of a primary care M.D. are not sick—I"m hoping that those who read this booklet will somehow be more inclined to help the patient even though the individual may not present with a temperature of 104. A sick person is one who seeks advice from another regarding his physical or emotional well being. Necessarily the complainer will seek educated help or sympathy from an empathetic ear. Practically, the sick one hopes for both. Every person you see in the office is seeking your ADVICE. They need not necessarily be in shock or extremis. You are not being hired as a God. The patient is asking for your advice. The patient may or may not heed your advice.

Before you begin you case studies, it has been said that THE SUFFERER WHO FRUSTRATES A KEEN THERAPIST BY FAILING TO IMPROVE IS ALWAYS IN DANGER OF MEETING PRIMITIVE HUMAN BEHAVIOR DISGUISED AS THERAPY!

It has also been said that MEDICINE MAY BE DEFINED AS THE ART OR SCIENCE OF KEEPING A PATIENT QUIET WITH FRIVILIOUS REASONS FOR HIS ILLNESS AND AMUSING HIM WITH REMEDIES GOOD OR BAD UNTIL NATURE KILLS OR CURES HIM.

Now to the case historys, ENJOY!!

Decubitus Ulcer

C.C. Nursing Home Patient with a broken hip who has bed sores (decubitus ulcers)

P.I Fell 2 months ago and sustained a fx hip—it was repaired and he was subsequently referred to a nursing home for further care.

F.H. Mother d. CVA

By System: Patient has prostate trouble and is incontinent.

P.H. No previous hospitalization—takes no medicine

P.X. A bony elderly man who smells of urine—is in a wet bed, and moves very little.

EENT R Pupil >L

CVR: BP 140/80

ABD : Scaphoid

Back: Silver dollar sized open sore over the coccyx.

DX: Bedsore (decubitus)

THE ONLY THING THAT WILL HELP IS TO KEEP THE WEIGHT OF THE BODY FROM JAMMING THE SORE AGAINST THE SHEET. This may be accomplished by getting the patient up, turning the patient on the side, or using a rubber ring. To clean the bedsore, offer whirlpool and a heat lamp. Perhaps one should consider an indwelling catheter since the patient is incontinent and the decubitus is constantly being bathed in urine. There are numerous lytic agents in a salve which help debride the wound and enhance healing but the MAIN TREATMENT REMAINS TO RELIEVE PRESSURE.

STROKE- FALL- FRACTURE

cc. headache, some trouble saying what comes in his mind. He was found on sidewalk outside his home—had fallen and had a broken hip with seen in ER

P.H. Has been on BP med for years

F.H. father died with a stroke and mother died age 56 with Ca colon

By systems—none significant

P.X. Pt slobbering and talking out of right side of mouth (left Facial paralysis) Pupils unequal

Chest clear. H.. reg BP 80/60

Abd- neg no masses or viscera palp

Ext.

Rt leg everted with painful movement of the right hip. Right arm flaccid (is this correct if the man is talking out of the right side of his mouth?)

DX FX hip—patient had a stroke and THEN FELL--- THIS IS QUITE COMMON

BITES

Many people come into an office with bites

1. Bug bites—best treated with some anesthetic cream to rub on and give the patient an antihistaminic for the itching.

2. Dog bites—These are serious in that the dog must be observed for the malady of rabies. The wound should be soaked in epsom salts--- The rule is to NEVER sew up a dog bit—if the laceration is severe— send to a surgeon. Antibiotics and a tetnus shot are the rule. The dog should be observed for 10 days in a wired pen or held by a secure chain. DO NOT USE A LEASH. If the dog is still alive after 10 days, it doesn't have rabies. If the dog dies or becomes ill,--take it to the Vet. DO NOT SHOOT THE DOG IN THE HEAD (many people do). 10 days is not too long to wait to begin rabies shots.

3. Human bites—These often get infected and are best treated with a tetanus shot and antibiotics plus soaking with epsom salts.

4. Rodent bites—mouse or rat or squirrel—usually do nothing except supportive care. give a booster tetanus shot and offer rabies vaccine after explaining the complications of that treatment.

5. Bat bite—They rarely bite, but the patient always thinks that they carry rabies. offer rabies treatment and give a tetanus shot.

6. Animal bites—horses, raccoon and etc. give a tetanus booster—soak and don't hesitate to call a vet regarding chances for rabies.

7. Patients should be advised regarding the danger of taking rabies shots. – encephalitis is a complication. Let the patient take the responsibility for making the decision on whether or not to take the rabies vaccine.

BE SURE that their decision is in writing or made before two witnesses.

Subarachnoid Hemorrhage

cc. Sudden severe headacke

P.H. never hospitalized. Married one year and takes BC pills—takes no other medicine. No history of recent trauma. No disasters or acute psychological trauma. She has a long history of headaches—she calls them migraines—frequently sick all day with cold towels to head and vomiting. Headaches are usually unilateral.

F.H. mother has migraines

PX   Patient has photophobia and pain behind the eyes. Keeps eyes closed. Her neck is slightly stiff, but not rigid. There is some nausea and she has vomited. Her sensorium is slightly disturbed.

Chest clear H.R. reg with noticeable bradycardia 60 (this happens with increased intrcranial pressure.) BP 110/70

abd: neg

Neuro: cranial nerves intact – no evidence of paralysis or neurological deficit

Differential

1. Migraine

2. Subarachnoid hemorrhage—(BC pills and history of headache make hemorrhage a good possibility)

LAB—CBC   wbc 18000 (Increase in wbc with blood on serosal surface)

Spinal tap—gross blood and increased protein with a normal sugar —normal sugar rules out bacteria—remember that they eat sugar!!

Final Diagnosis—Subarachnoid hemorrhage

THE PATIENT WHO HAS FREQUENT HEADACHES SHOULD PROBABLY NOT TAKE BC PILLS

Cancer Breast

CC. Pain and swelling in the right armpit

PH para 1 grav 1 did not nurse child no previous serious illness. Takes extrogen for hot flashes—(two conditions extrogen and not nursing inc the chances of ca breast.)

FH nothing significant except one sister had ca breast (another risk factor)

PX WDWN afro-american who is slightly obese and in no acute distress

EENT neg no ant or post cervical nodes and no supraclavicular nodes

Axillae—Multiple nodes in the right axilla clearly felt and not movable— these are tender to palpation. (matted and not freely movable is the key)

Chest clear to a and p

Breast: Right breast demonstrates a mass 2 cm in diameter in the upper outer quadrant. (UPPER OUTER IS THE BIG DANGER ZONE))

Lab—Mammogram shows mass suspicious for malignancy

Chest x-ray normal

Disposition: Refer to surgeon

Overmedicated

cc. too tired to get up

P.I. began with a fx leg 6 months ago—this was followed by PT and repeated exams by physicians when she just didn't do well. She was slow to recover from surgery and never did SNAP OUT of her dilemma

Repeated CBC's were normal. After the cast was removed—more PT was accomplished, but the patient continued to lay in bed.

P.H. always active, but recently son became divorced which caused her some loss of sleep

Soc Hist.   husband is a doctor who didn't pay her much attention to her illness

PX completely healthy looking

EENT neg

BP 145/85

All physical finding neg except patient appeared somnolent.

CLOSER QUESTIONING REVEALS THAT THE PATIENT HAD HAD SLEEPING PILLS FROM THE ORTHOPEDIC SURGEON—FROM HER HUSBAND, AND FROM HER

PRIMARY CARE DOCTOR—THEY WERE ALL DIFFERENT AND SHE WAS TAKING THEM ALL

DX. OVERMEDICATION

Treatment—remove medication

Tic Doloreaux

C.C. pain in the face

P.I. Began 2 weeks ago and is increasingly severe. Pain is sharp—knife
–like and comes in paroxysms. It is triggered by cold food, cold air,
brushing the teeth. It is a TERRIBLE PAIN – always in the same area
and is unbearable.

P.X. WDWN   caucasian female not acutely ill but afraid to talk for
fear it will bring on pain

EENT: cranial nerves intact – pupils round and equal

Chest clear-- heart rate regular   BP   120/808

Abdomen negative

THERE IS A PAUCITY OF POSITIVE FINDINGS

IMPRESSION TRIGEMINAL NEURALGIA

(TIC DOLOREAUX)

DIFFERENTIAL

1. Rule out tooth or sinus abscess

Treatment : Many of these people will require narcotics. Begin with dilantin, then try simpl;e analgesics or narcotics if needed—later try Tegretal—If no help, refer to neurosurgeon who will strip the nerve.

Gynecomastia

C.C.   One breast is larger than the other and is tender.

P.I. Young man is being teased by middle-school classmates because his breasts are big. This young man finally came to his father who brought him to the clinic. (the father is usually in attendance)

P.H. No serious illnesses. Has been on no medication. Feels good. Appetite hearty—voice has been changing recently

F.H. Not significant,

D.X. Gynecomastia

Discussion: It is important to examine the testicles after explaining that a tumor of the testicle may cause this. I have never found a tumor, but after you don't find a tumor, you may explain that when the hormones are coming to light that the male and female hormones are vieing for dominance—the male always wins, but in the interim, some female hormone excess may make the breasts or breast large and sore. This will all go away in a few weeks!! Reassure the patient and the father that all is well.

Salivary Gland Stone

C.C.   Swelling right side of face

P.I.   Began one week ago when right side of face beneath and in front of the ear began to swell. –especially after eating,-- then swelling would recede until another meal.

P.H. non- informing.

F. H.   normal

By systems—neg

Physical exam.---WDWN   colored 40 year old who appears well

EENT: Stenson"s duct, which is opposite the 2nd molar on the right is inflammed with obvious white object protruding from the orifice. This "stone" was expressed with the fingers by gently squeezing just behind the orifice. The duct then bled slightly.

Final diagnosis—SALIVARY STONE OCCLUDING STENSON"S DUCT

Differential—mumps (how does this duct appear in mumps?—look up)

One can usually feel this stone by gently having the index finger over the duct and the thumb outside the cheek!

Hemospermia

C.C. Blood in sperm

P.H. Wife noticed blood in semen on two occasions. She has had hysterectomy and is not sure from intercourse.

P.H. Has had no previous serious illnesses. Never in bed over one week (a good question to ferret illness) Takes no medication (blood thinners)

F.H. negative—father living and well and still working full time as a farmer.

By systems—all normal except G.U. Has been getting up at nite to urinate—occasional burning with urination.

Soc History: In the navy and comes home every 6 months. Has been having intercourse 3-4 times a day.

P.X. Healthy man not acutely ill

All exams are normal except on exquisitly tender prostate.

Differential:

1. Prostatitis

2. malignancy of seminal vesicles or testes or prostate

Lab 1. PSA slightly elevated (psa is not a specific test for malignancy, but can be elevated with prostatitis or massage of the prostate such as riding a bicycle)

Treatment

1. Intercourse at a reasonable rate

2. 10 days course of antibiotics

3. call or return if symptoms persist

Hemospermia is a frequent complaint and is usually due to prostatitis— It is almost never a symptom of serious disease.

Angina

CC. PAIN IN CHEST

P.I. HAS BEEN NOTICING PAIN IN MID-STERNAL AREA WITH EXERTION. I.E. CLIMBING STAIRS OR HURRYING. THE PAIN STOPS WITH REST—IT DOES NOT RADIATE TO ARMS OR BACK

P.H. KNOWN DIABETIC ON 36 U NPH

F.H.   FATHER DIED WITH DIABETES

MOTHER LIVING AND WELL AGE 80

ONE BROTHER WITH SUGAR AND ANGINA PECTORIS

BY SYSTEMS; NO PROBLEMS EXCEPT CVR; PAIN IN CHEST IS EXERTIONAL AND RELIEVED BY NITROGLYCERINE TABLETS UNDER THE TONGUE –GIVEN TO HER BY A FRIEND

LAB;   CBC NORMAL, EKG NORMAL, CHEST X-RAY NORMAL

STRESS TEST—STRONGLY POSITIVE

DISPOSITION; REFERRAL TO CARDIOLOGIST FOR CATH WHICH DEMONSTATED 3 VESSEL DISEASE, SEVERE, REQUIRING OPEN HEART SURGERY

Diabetes, Adult Onset

C.C. urinating too much

P.I. Began 2 months ago and has been getting progressively worse. Now gets up every two hours to pass copious amounts.

P.H. had " Brights disease" as a child—(look this up)

By Systems. G.U. some difficulty starting urine early am. Has noticed increased thirst.

P.X. Well looking white male in no distress. EEN T- neg. eyegrounds reveal a few flame hemorrhages—(an important finding)

Chest clear to A&P-=-normal breath sounds. Abdomen soft—no masses or viscera palpable. EXT.—1 plus edema with mod severe varicosities.

DIFFERENTIAL DIAGNOSIS

1.   prostatism

2.   diabetes mellitus

3.   X-S caffeine as in coffee, tea, or cokes

4.   taking diuretics

5.   Diabetes insipitus

6.   Renal failure

NOTE; he should have been asked if he was taking any medicine. He also wasn't asked if he used caffeine—he wasn't questioned about wt loss or gain. A good question is not "have you lost any weight?" –but the question should be—"What did you weigh 6 months ago?"

LAB WORK—chem 12 and psa revealed a fasting blood sugar of 450—all else was normal , i.e., psa, bun, cbc and etc.

FINAL DIAGNOSIS—Diabetes Mellitus –adult onset

Appendicitis

cc. pain R.L.Q. in a 30 year old male

P.I. Began 2 days ago with nagging pain. Now hurts to cough—has severe pain in the belly and isn't hungry. He is running a low grade temp.

P.H. never sick before—never hospitalized—never in bed for over one week (these are good questions to ask in obtaining a history)

By systems: EENT – neg

CVR – has recently had a cold and sore throat (red herring)

G.I. – diahrrea for 3 days (red herring) usually are constipated

G.U. – some burning with urination (red herring) can get this with a fever or with peritoneal irritation.

Physical exam:

Temp 99.8 in a WDWN; white male who is walking somewhat bent over and guards his stomach

EENT—neg

Chest clear BP normal:

ABDOMEN—board like abdomen with no bowel sounds.

Genetalia –neg

Lab—WBC 18000 with a shift to the left (inc. neurtophils)

THIS IS A RUPTURED APPENDIX

It has often been said that if you can diagnose appendicitis—you can diagnose anything. Notice the roadblocks, i e , diahrrea, burning with urination , low temperature, and etc. PICK OUT the main symnptoms and pursue the diagnosis

Cancer Prostate

cc. Pain in back—severe

P.I. began 2 weeks ago when he lifted his 3 year old grandson—no previous back trouble.

P.H. Hard working laborer who has never had a serious illness

F.H. non-informing

By systems: Occasionally sob and some difficulty starting urine stream in early am. Loss of libido

P.X. well nourished muscular elderly man who doesn't apperar to be sick

EENT—neg CVR clear—heart rate reg—BP 140/86

ABD: normal no viscera or masses palpable Rectal: Prostate hard (stone –like) on the left

Differential

1. Arthritis

2. Fx spine , pathological

3. Pulled muscle

4. Bone lesion

Order :

x-rays of back—all came back normal

Bone scan—positive for widespread metastasis

Lab: PSA—36

Diagnosis Ca prostate with mets to spine and pathological fracture.

Gout

cc. painful urination

PI started yesterday when he noticed blood in the urine—goes frequently to urinate and it is very painful—hot and burns

PH   no previous problems

never hospitalized

takes no medicine

no trauma

FH   normal except father has gouty arthritis

BY systems   neg

PX   EENT negative—patient is afebrile

Chest clear to a and p   BP 120/80

Abd   neg—LS&K not palp (no tenderness to percussion over kidneys as is often found with any acute kidney problem) no peripheral edema and prostate and genitalia are normal

Order:

1. urine—loaded with blood

2. uric acid (father had gout) This was elevated

3. IVP—which showed small calculus on Right

Treatment: Give pain medication—usually a narcotic and STRAIN ALL URINE AND SEND STONE FOR ANALYSIS

This stone was recovered and was a uric acid stone

Final DX Gout with ureteral stone

Headaches

C.C.   CHRONIC HEADACHES

This discussion is not intended as a "sine qua non" for the diagnosis of headache, but perhaps will give you a starting place when the patient presents with headache.

KEEP DETAILED NOTES RE ANSWERS TO QUESTIONS, IMPRESSIONS AND ETC AS NO ONE CAN USUALLY MAKE A DIAGNOSIS OF THE CAUSE OF HEADACHE IN ONE VISIT.

1. Location of headache. Unilateral (migraine) Behind the eyes (eyestrain or inc. intracranial pressure) vortex of head (usually nothing important)

2. Does anything aggravate the headache such as light (migraine) hay fever or pollen increase or odors of perfume or other noxious substancers?

3. When did the headaches begin? With marriage, with inlaws moving in our out,with tension, with new glasses, with a cold , with an

infection, with unfaithful husband or wife, with drainage from sinus?

4. What relieves the headache? narcotics, aspirin, bed rest, sex, vacations.

5. Are there associated symptoms such as an aura (migraine), nausea, vomiting or stiff neck

6. Is there a past history of trauma or have they had a diagnosis of arthritis of the spine?

7. Remember that headache is a prominent symptom of encephalitis, meningitis, typhoid, and any FUO or acute elevation of temperatuare.

8. Environmental causes such as gas leakage in the house or other causes such as pine trees or dusty roads.

9. What has been your previous diagnoses. ? LET THE PATIENT TALK ABOUT THEIR HEADACHE.

10. Is the patient after narcotics? Is the patient knowledgeable about the various common treatments for headache? Does the patient recite about drugs as if he or she published the PDR ? Be on the lookout for addicts.

The physical exam:

Does the patient look well? Does the patient evidence weight loss? Do a complete EENT exam and check all of the cranial nerves. Check the fundus for papilloedema and the retinae for hemorrhages. The BP should be checked and re-chcked. As you see the patient and become acquainted , you may want a CT scan of the head, a sed rate, cbc, urine, and routine chem tests.

Black Stools

cc. my BM's are black and I am weak

PH how long has this been—2days. "This is the first time—ever" Has been taking iron because she has felt tired. Also takes pepto-bismol for a burning in her stomach

PH never hospitalized—works as a maid and has 4 small children at home. She is not married

By systems—all neg—she has lost no weight and eats fast foods. She smokes 2 pkg per day

PX completely normal abd—the rectal reveals coal black-tarry-sticky-smelly stool on glove.

Lab Hb 10 otherwise neg except for hemastix on stool was positive

DIFFERENTIAL;

1.. BLACK STOOLS DUE TO IRON (NOT TARRY, NOT STICKY, NOT FETID ODOR) THESE STOOLS ARE USUALLY CHARCHOL STOOLS AND NOT JET BLACK

2. BLACK STOOLS DUE TO PEPTO- BISMOL (USUALLY BLACK, BUT AGAIN NOT TARRY OR STICKY OR FOUL SMELLING AND CHOCOLATE RATHER THAN COAL BLACK)

3. Black stools due to blood—low HB and stools are fetid, sticky and tarry referred to X-ray where a gastric ulcer was demonstrated gastric ulcers are best referred because of the possibility of malignancy

PEOPLE WHO BLEED SLOWLY CAN FUNCTION ON A HB OF 6 OR 7 WHEREAS AN ACUTE BLEED REDUCING THE HB PRECIPTIOUSLY TO 6-7 WILL PUT THE PATIENT DOWN

Cellulitis Hand

cc. sore armpit

PI. got up this am and noticed "kernel" in right armpit which was sore—no chills or fever

PH neg not taking any med. no previous hospitalization

FH neg both parents living and well. no familial disease

PX normal looking young lad who does not appear ill

Afebrile, BP 110/80 Pulse 76 resp 20

The right upper ext reveals a splinter in his palm which he has been trying to get out for 2 days with a "sterilized" safety pen. Further exam reveals red streaks up the forearm (lymphatics) Right axilla has multiple nodes which are painful—the largest is 2 cm in diameter.

Lab—urine to R.O. diabetes

DX cellulitis hand with regional adenopathy treatment—soaks with epsom salts and antibiotic

Cancer Stomach with Sentinel Node

CC. STOMACH TROUBLE

P.I. APPETITE HAS LESSENED AND HE HAS LOST #10 IN THE LAST MONTH. HAS HAD ULCER PAINS RELIEVED BY ROLAIDS. STOOLS HAVEN'T CHANGED IN COLOR AND HE HAS HAD NAUSEA, BUT NO VOMITING.

P[H—ONE PREVIOUS HOSPITALIZATION FOR APPENDICITIS

FH. MOTHER DIED WITH STROKE

ONE BROTHER DIED CANCER COLON

FATHER DIED BRAIN TUMOR

BY SYSTEMS; NOTHING SIGNIFICANT

PX

GAUNT LOOKING CAUCASIAN WHO LOOKS PALE AND CHR. ILL.

EENT—NEG EXCEPT HAS A LARGE TENDER SUPRA-
CLAVICULAR MODE ON THE LEFT SIDE. THIS MEASURES
1 1/2 cm. AND IS SYMETRICAL AND HARD

LAB—ORDER CXR AND CBC AND STOMACH X-RAY

BUT WE ALREADY KNOW THAT T HIS IS CANCER OF THE
STOMACH WITH A LARGE SENTINEL NODE WHICH IS
SUPRA-CLAVICULAR ON THE LEFT—PATHOGNOMIC!!!

Spermatocele

C.C. I have a knot on my testicle

P.I. Patient has noticed this knot on his testicle for about 6 months. He has been reading and is afraid he has a cancer. The knot is not larger—there is no tenderness. Sexual function has been normal. He has had no chills or fever and feels fine.

P.H. Takes no medication. Has never been hospitalized. Denies trauma to the testicle.

F.H. Mother and Father both living and well. "My family is a healthy bunch"!

By Systems: Entirely normal

Work History: This man is a machinist who does moderately heavy lifting.

Soc History: Active in sports. Plays baseball and golf

P.X. Athletic young man who appears well.

EENT: neg

CVR: neg

ABD: L,S, and K not palp—no masses or viscera palp. No tenderness. no nodes in groin.

No evidence of hernia.

EXT: negative

Genitalia: Normal appearing. Rt and Left Testicles are a normal size. On the pole of the right testicle there is a freely movable, rather hard, pea sized mass which is not tender. No other finding.

Rectal: Mucosa smooth—prostate soft and normal size.

IMPRESSION: This is a spermatocele

Discussion: This mass is connected to but not a part of the testicle. It is freely movable, not tender. Spermatoceles are a dime a dozen and the treatment is simple reassurance. If this becomes large or uncomfortable, the patient can return and consider surgical removal. I can't remember this happening.

BPH with Chr. Urinary Retention

C.C. "I am having trouble with passing my water"!

P.I. Began 3 months ago when patient noticed he was urinating frequently and only small amounts. Today, so far, he has been unable to urinate.

P.H. Has been taking stomach medicine for the last 4 months. His Dr. told him he might have an ulcer. (What is the effect of an atropine-like drug on bladder or prostate?)

By Systems

All neg except

G.I. Has been having discomfort in lower abdomen—midline over the pubis

F.H. Father had prostate trouble

P.X. Healthy looking elderly male in acute distress with inability to urinate—sweat on his brow and pain in lower abdomen

CVR: B.P. elevated 190/100 HR regular. chest clear

ABD: Palp mass over the pubis—soft, tender (probably bladder)

Ext: negative

Rectal: mucosa clear—smooth mucosa—very large smooth prostate which is not hard

D.X. This is acute urinary retention probably due to BPH

The treatment is to introduce a catheter in order to allow the bladder to empty. If the bladder is emptied quickly, the patient might go into shock. The catheter should be clamped and release 30 cc of urine every 5- 10 minutes until the bladder is empty. Then referral to a urologist for definitive care.

Gout

C.C. Painful right toe

P.I. Came on suddenly—this is the first time to have a sore toe. Awakened in the middle of the night with the toe throbbing and red. – so painful that EVEN THE BED CLOTHES MAKE IT HURT.

P.H. has had one bout of kidney stones and passed the stone two years ago. The stones were not analyzed. (It is important to send any stone to the lab for identification—if it is a uric acid stone—the diagnosis is definite.) No other serious illnesses—Elbows occasionally bother him— No history of trauma to the toe (don't be caught without asking the patient about obvious trauma—remember that the patient frequently knows the diagnosis and is testing your ability)

P.X., EENT—tophi in ear (look up this physical finding) The exam is negative except for the right foot—the great toe is swollen and red near the end of the first metatarsal (base of toe) There are no red streaks. The toe is exquisitly TENDER—do not touch unless you want a mad patient.

D.X. Gout

Treatment—colchicine and symptomatic treatment

Cancer Pancreas

cc. yellow skin

P.I. Patient noticed that his eyes were yellow one week ago. Now skin is yellow and he itches all over.

P.H. no previous hospitalization

takes no meds

Has been around no unusual chemicals

drinks 2 shots scotch daily and has for years

F.H. not significant

By Systems—yellow skin has been progressively worse. Now his urine is quite dark and his bowel movements are clay colored—(indicating complet obstruction of bile)

G.I. appetite fair—no weight loss—no pain or discomfort in the abdomen

P.X. A well nourished middle aged man who is quite yellow , but otherwise appears hail and hearty. With the exception of jaundice, the physical exam was completely within normal limits—the abdomen was soft. no masses or viscera were palpable and there was no tenderness.

Lab—cbc normal,--urine positive for bile. chem 12—elevated bilirubin—
sed rate normal.

Diagnosis: PAINLESS PROGRESSIVE JAUNDICE IS
PATHOGNOMONIC OF CANCER OF THE HEAD OF THE
PANCREAS!

Cholecystitis

C.C. Pain in the RUQ

P.I. pain has been off and on for the last 2 years. Seems to occur after meals—especially if the meals are greasy such as pork chops and gravy—Occasionally happens after eating ice cream. Now has nausea and some vomiting

P.H. Has had appendix out and 3C-sections. (Gall bladder disease is much more frequent in women who are multipara)

F.H. Mother had stomach trouble which was never diagnosed. Father had gout and one brother had gout. (what stomach or kidney problems occur with gout?)

By Systems—EENT—someone told her that her eyes were yellow G.I. stools are clay colored (no bile) G.U. Urine is dark (bile)

P.X. A middle aged woman who is yellow—i.e. sclera and skin—(when questioned she said that she has severe itching of the skin and this happens with bile deposit in the skin) Chest clear to A & P She has a noticeable bradycardia (this occurs with jaundice) ABD: exquisite tenderness RUQ—no masses or viscera are palpable. (If the G.B. is palpable, it is distended and this is almost pathognomonic of malignancy of the biliary system)

Impression:

1. Acute G.B.

2. R.O. malignancy of the biliary system

Order sonogram of the abdomen—this revealed multiple small stones in the gall bladder and the patient was referred to a surgeon.

Common Cold

cc nose running

P.I. Patient states that this is the worst cold I have ever had. She recently visited her daughter in California and 2 days after returning by air suddenly began sneezing and now rose runs all the time and she has trouble sleeping. Her daughter has a cat and she has been told she is allergic to house dust.

P.H. Has been in the hospital for G.B. surgery, appendix, hysterectomy, and carpal tunnel syndrome. Has been taking benadryl—no help!!

Family H. Husband smokes and she is allergic to smoke

P.X. Well looking female who has a runny nose Temp 99

EENT conjunctiva red—throat slightly red with some clear drainage in post pharynx

no nodes

Chest clear and a and p. No Wheezing BP 130/75 H.R. reg

abd- neg ext neg

THIS IS RATHER TYPICAL OF A SIMPLE COMMON COLD FOR WHICH LITTLE CAN BE DONE. THE PATIENT WILL EXPECT TREATMENT—THEREFORE GIVE ASCRIPTIN OR SOME EXOTIC ASPIRIN THAT HAS A FANCY NAME. CAUTION THE PATIENT THAT IF A FEVER GREATER THAN 100 OCCURS—CALL BACK

Pink Eye (Conjunctivitis)

C.C. My eyelids were stuck together when I awakened this am.

P.I. Has not been bothered with this before. Eye itched last night before she went to bed. Has had no foreign body in the eye. Has been using no eyedrops.—this just came "out of the blue".

P.H. Para 2, Grav 2. otherwise never hospitalized. Takes no medication.

F.H. Not significant except mother a diabetic.

By Systems: nothing significant. She tests her blood about every 6 mo since her mother is a diabetic and she has always been normal.

Soc Hist: House wife with children age 6 and 8. A housefull of kids most of the time and 2 days ago had a visitor with a sore eye.

PX. Well looking lady with a red right eye which has crusts on the eyelids.

EENT: The right conjunctiva is inflamed and very red. The pupils are round and equal.

The iris appears to be normal and the ant chambers are clear. Funduscopic is entirely normal. The eyelashs are crusted and there is a creamy exudate in the corner of the eye.

D.X. This is CONJUNCTIVITIS or "pink eye"

Discussion: This malady responds readily to local antibiotics which are usually dispensed in an optic cream. Both eyes are usually treated as this is a highly contagious condition. Usually the patient is instructed to wear colored glasses as photophobia can be a problem. The family should be cautioned re using the same towels and etc. and keeping the hands clean by frequent washing. This condition responds readily and the eye should be greatly iimproved in 48 hours. Meantime, the child must not go to school.

Decubitus Heel

C.C. Ulcers on both heels

P.I. This patients has been in a nursing home for 6 month. This admission followed hospitalization for a stroke. She has been bedfast since admission.

P.H. She is on high BP medicine and takes lasix. She has had no operations or previous hospitalization.

P.X. A poorly nourished , thin female who looks as if she had been in a concentration camp. She is lifeless and speaks with difficulty . She looks chronically ill.

EENT: Bil cataracts—otherwise neg.

CVR: Chest clear to A/P   H.R, Reg—no murmurs. Rate 80   Resp Rate 20

ABD: Scaphoid—no masses or viscera palpable

EXT: 2 large 2 cm. rounded black areas which are draining on both heels. These areas are not particularly uncomfortable and are not painful to the touch.

DX: DECUTITUS ULCERS OF THE HEELS

This never should have happened. The main thing is to ANTICIPATE THE PROBLEM-use heel protectors, cream to soften the skin, and prop the feet on pillows to prevent constant pressure on the heels. If, in spite of prophylaxis, the patient develops decubitus. then the treatment is whirlpool and relief of the pressure.

Lacerated Tendon

C.C. Laceration of the finger

P.I. Patient was opening a can of beans when her hand slipped and she cut her left index (ist) finger on the volar side.

P.H. Takes no medicine, and never hospitalized

P.X. Limited to the hand—Exam reveals 1 1/2 cm. gash on the palmer surface of the index finger. On close exam, one can identify a partially lacerated tendon. This is noticeable when asking the patient to flex and extend the finger.

Treatment:

NEVER, NEVER try to repair any tendon. This is for experts and the patient should be referred immediatel;y. The temptation will be great, BUT refer the patient for any tendon injury.

Hypothroidism

CC: Dry Skin

P.I. Patient has noticed that her skin is flaky and dry over the last 6 months.

P.H. Has never been hospitalized and takes no medicine. She is overly tired and has gained about 40# in the last 4 months.

By Systems:

CVR takes her pulse frequently and it is always slow

Endo: She is cold all the time and doesn't sweat at all anymore.

P.X. This is a heavy set woman who has a thick speech (mush in her mouth) . She has a bull dog appearance and an apathetic (blank look) face and is obviously mentally dull.

EENT—neg

CVR—Heart rate reg 60. B.P 130/75 Chest Clear to A/P

ABD – pendulous—no viscera palpable

EXT: 2 + pitting edema pre-tibial surface.

Differential

1. Simple Obesity

2. Possible Hypothroidism

Lab: CBC – Urine—normal Throid Panel including TSH and T4. This revealed hypothroidism! What would you expect the thyroid panel to reveal in a hypothyroism?

THIS IS A CLASSIC HYPOTHYROID—ONE NEED NOT PRESENT WITH ALL OF THE SYMPTOMS—maybe only tiredness, obesity, dry skin, bradycardia or apathetic look. Think of hypothyroidism as a motor which is idling.. Think of hyperthyroidism as a motor which is reved up. i.e. boundless energy, skinny, moist skin, anxious look, and tachycardia

Pneumonitis

cc SOB

PI began with a cold 4 days ago. —runny nose, sneezing and sore throat. Progressed on to a cold and today coughed up red blood—Feels good-No complaints other than SOB

PH Has been having trouble with joints and 5 days ago saw a rheumatologist who put him on cortisone for 10 days—otherwise has never had a sick day

FH mother and father and 4 sibling living and well

PX BP 140/90   Temp 98   Resp 30

Well looking , spry, middle aged man who is sob

EENT—neg   Chest reveals absent breath sounds on the right lower. Dull to percussion

ABD neg

EXT neg

Differential

1. Pneumania

2. pleural effusion

Lab CBC normal

chest x-ray --lower lobe on right shows complete consolidation—i.e. lobar pneumonia

DX sever pneumonia

CORTISONE WILL MASK SYMPTOMS,--MASK LAB—MASK TEMP ELEVATION AND GIVE THE PATIENT A FALSE SENSE OF WELL BEING

Erythema Nodosum

cc. sore legs

PI   sore spots about the size of a quarter occurred 3 week ago—these aren't leaving—in fact, there are getting worse. At the same time , his joints began to ache, but no swelling. Temp elevation to 101 at night and low grade thru day.

PH had a cold one mo ago and treated this with OTC medication. He can't remember the drug.

PX

WDWN caucasian with temp 99 oral   BP 110/80 P. 100

Chest clear—dry cough

skin OK except pre-tibial, red, swollen, hot, tender nodules 1-2 cm in diameter. These are multiple—easily defined, but do no coalesce.

Differential

1. fixed drug reaction

2. erythema nodosum

Lab CBC

wbc 11000 with a shift to left and no inc in eosinophils

Discussion: This is a difficult differential which is largely academic. The treatment is with steroids—fixed drug reactions are usually not so limited to the pre-tibial surfaces and drug reactions are usually accompanied by eosinophils. Drug reactions usually abate after3-4 weeks whereas erythema nodosum hangs on for months. This case most clearly demonstrates erythema nodosum.

Lymphatic Leukemia

cc. Rash

PI Rash began on legs three days ago—doesn't itch and seems to be spreading. Mostly on shins and lower legs. No history of trauma,. This is bilateral---

PH takes no medicine. Takes no OTC drugs. (patients usually don't count medicines that they can pick up at the drug store as drugs)

FH not significant

By systems—not significant

PX exam of conjunctiva reveals small petechial hemorrhages –Chest clear BP 130/80 ABD. neg LS&K not palpable

ext—Bilateral petechial hemorrhages on both shins—mod severe

Differential

1. Low or abnormal platelets

2. Drug reaction

3. Blood Dyscrasia

Lab CBC revealed WBC 30,000 with 80% lymphocytes

DX early lymphocytic leukemia

NOSEBLEED

Sudden vomiting of bright red blood

This began suddenly and the patient called the nurse to the bedside—
The amount of vomitus was about one cup—fresh blood

PH Patient was in nursing home for custodial care. Had had high BP
for years and was taking lo-pressor 50 mgm bid.

The nurse reported that the patient complained of no pain in the abdomen
and that palpation of the abdomen revealed no tenderness BP 220/100
The patient was freightened . Pulse 120

THE DOCTOR DID NOT SEE THE PATIENT AND ALL
ORDERS WERE ACCOMPLISHED BY PHONE

Stat CBC Hb 11.2 normal differential

Stat Chest X-ray—normal

Stat upper GI –normal

The patient vomited again—about a cup of fresh blood

The doctor then visited the patient –first saying "Just how do you feel"
The patient replied that "I think my nose has stopped bleeding"

DEMONSTRATING THE VALUE OF A CAREFUL HISTORY

Parkinson's Disease

C.C. hands shake

P.I. began 2-3 years ago and has been getting progressively worse. One hand worse than the other. Bothers him most when he is trying to do something.

P.H. No serious accidents of hospitalizations. Had TIA two years ago and has been taking aspirin daily

F.H. father had same tremors—Mother died with diabetes—no sibling

By systems—all okay except muscular-skeleton—Walks slightly bent forward and hurries as if trying to catch up with himself. ARMS DON'T SWING AS HE WALKS.

Physical Exam elderly man who is confused as to time and place with a MASK like face.

EENT Neg

Chest—clear to and auscultation and percussion Heart rate reg BP 140/90

Abdomen—neg

Extremeties: doesn't swing arms when walking—walks bent forward and tends to lurch forward—Pill rolling with right index finger and thumb (this was the old pharmaceutical method of mixing pills—they rolled the ingredients between their thumb and forefinger to create a ball) Has a tremor especially of the right hand which is made worse by trying to eat or pick up an object.

Diagnosis—PARKINSONS DISEASE

TREATMENT USUALLY L-DOPA

Differential—familial tremor—familial tremor is hereditary and usually is not an intention tremor. (Look up intention tremor) The patient doesn't lurch. arms swing and it is helped by inderol.

Bell's Palsy

CC I may have had a stroke and I can't spit

P.I. began one day ago when awakened and found mouth drawn.— slobbered when trying to drink and can't sip thru a straw. family all sure this is a stroke.

P.H. no significant illnesses—has never had high blood pressure

By systems EENT some pain behind the ear on the affected side (this is typical) generally feels good—no headache—no chills or fever.

Physical Exam healthy appearing young white female whose face is drawn on the left. The wrinkles in the forehead are missing on the left. and the lip on the left is sagging—patient can't smile or wrinkle forehead There is unilateral facial parazlysis of the facial nerve—can't whistle— face mask like on the left

BP 120/80

Differential

1. CVA

2. Bell's Palsy (7TH NERVE PARALYSIS)

Final DX. This is truly a bell's palsy—she has pain behind the ear—no other signs of paralysis except 7th nerve. she has a feeling of well being

treatment—watchful waiting. This usually lasts approximately 2 weeks and patient should be warned that occasionally, ie, rarely, it will persist. Also , it may recur.

CHF with Auricular Fib

C.C. ankles swollen

P.I. began one week ago!

getting progressively worse—feet are tender and both ankles are swelling—no prevcious problems with the feet

P.H. High BP for years (blacks often have intractable BP) She is on lopressor (this can cause edema) She knows that many doctors have told her that her heart rate is irregular.

F.H.   Father died with dropsy (the old folks call CHF dropsy)

      Mother died with CVA

By systems. CVR: has recently developed a cough and notices shortness of breath when bending, stooping, or climbing stairs. Now uses 2-3 pillows to elevate her head when sleeping. No pain in chest

P.X. 65 year old who is obviously very short of breath

EENT neg : pupils round and equal (what if pupils are unequal—stroke—trauma—operation?) look this up!!

CVR: BP 180/110 Heart rate irregular irregularity with a pulse deficit of 40 (pulse deficit is the difference between the apical and radial rate) Lungs have moist rales in both bases. The abdominal exam is neg except the liver is down 2 fingers.

EXT—2 plus pitting edema

Impression CHF with auricular fibrillation

Treatment—patient should have low salt diet.—ace inhibitors and a diuretic and be followed closely for intended improvement. Since the patient knows that her heart has been irregular for years, no attempt should be made to cause the rythym to be regular—recent onset fibrillation should be referred to a cardiologist for attempts at conversion.

Lymphoma

C.C. Itching skin

P.I. has been noticing that her skin is itching ESPECIALLY AFTER TAKING A HOT BATH. she has noticed no color changes of skin (jaundice). no rash—the itching does not occur at night (pinworms) and she notices no itching due to clothing change (wool)

P.H. Para II, Grav II

By systems G.I. 10# weight loss in 6 mo, but has been on a diet. (I am always suspicious of weight loss because diets, in general, don't work for any length of time)

B.M.'s okay Has recently noticed tiredness especially in the afternoon!

Physical Exam:

No positive physical findings—Attention was given to the skin which showed no evidence of parasites. There was no jaundice. No bradycardia (occurs with jaundice)

Blood Studies – Chem 12 normal. Sed rate elevated to 29 CBS revealed a Hb of 10.5 with an Fe def type anemia.

Chest X-ray—bilateral hilar enlargement suggestive of lymphoma

This patient was referred to a pulmonologist who made a dx of early lynmphoma

ITCHING OF THE BODY—ESPECIALLY AFTER A HOT BATH—IN THE FACE OF A PAUCITY OF PHYSICAL FINDING ALWAYS SHOULD BRING LYMPHOMA TO MIND

(now you can worry about itching)

Pityriasis Rosea

C.C. Rash all over the body

P.I. this started about one week ago—gradually spreading over trunk an back. It began with a large area of dermatitis in a patch on the chest wall (3 cm by 3 cm) This has been named a "herald patch" and is frequently found in this condition. There has been no chills or fever and very little itching.

P.H. no serious diseases. has no history of V.D.. (Syphilis frequently manifests itself as a rash) She recently has gotten a divorce (old docs taught that this usually happened after a catastrophy or major event such as a house burning down, a divorce, or a death in the immediate family)

P.X. Limited to the skin shows practically no lesions on "ANYPLACE THAT SHOWS' i.e., hands and face. No lesions on palm (secondary syphilis) no mouth lesions. The lesions are small, flakey and do not coalasce. Furthermore,. the lesions follow the lines of clevage on the breast, abdomen, trunk, and on the back.

IMPRESSION:

PITYRIASIS ROSEA

Rule out syphilis

This is a self limited disease—usually lasts about 2 week. Oatmeal baths help!

PVC's

C.C. My heart is missing beats and turning over in my chest.

P.I. Began 3 months ago and now she notices it quite ofter—especially after eating.

P.H. Para 4, Gravida 5 who is a housewife. Never seriously ill. Takes aspirin occasionally for headache.

By Systems

EENT: neg

CVR: no cough or SOB. No edema. no pains in chest

G.I. Some wt gain. Drinks 8-10 cups coffee per day.

M.J. No findings

M.N. Contemplating divorce. Husband having an affair.

D.X. PVC's (extrasystoles)

P,X. Entirely within normal limits B.P. 125/75 HR reg . no murmurs or thrills. No extra beats heard

Lab: CBC, urine, EKG   all normal

Discussion: These PVC's are most commonly caused by caffeine, coffee, tea, cokes, chocolate, or OTC medicines containing caffeine. They can also be caused by stress. They are innocuous and the patient shoul;d be reassured that a heart attack is not imminent. Modify eating and drinking habits and help the patient to cope with stress by suggesting family counseling.

Herpes Zoster

C.C. Painful rib cage on the left for one week

P.I. pain has been progressively worse for one week—now aspirin and ibuprofen do not help and this is the worst pain I have ever had—even worse than labor pains.. It doesn't hurt to take a deep breath. No symptoms of a cold. Has been running a low grade fever—99.6. No history of trauma. Pain is severe and extends from the front around to the back.

P.H. nothing like this previously takes no medication. recently returned from a two week stay in florida and has a nice tan. (herpes is frequently precipitated by ultra violet light.)

Physical Exam:

well looking male who does not appear acutely or chronically ill.

Chest clear to a&p—there is a small area the size of 1/2 dollar posteriorly at the level of the 6th rib which is broken out with vesicles—some of which have bursted. Vesicles (blisters) are wee to the size of a pea. they are red and angry looking. Physical exam is otherwise negative

IMPRESSION   Herpes Zoster

Treatment—prednisone in selected cases. ?? ?? ?? Analgesics—otherwise the treatment is symptomatic. The patient should be alerted to the fact that these frquently break out for two weeks—are very painful and may continue to hurt for week, months, or years after the attack. Also they do recur.

Read about Herpes vaccine

LABYRINTHITIS

P.I. Has been noticing increasing bouts of dizziness for several months. It is aggravated by moving the head. No headaches. Eyesight the same. occasional nausea with the dizziness, but no vomiting. no weight loss. not seeing double.

P.H. No previous hospitalization. never in bed over one week (a good question for ferreting out past illness) Takes a lot of alka seltzer for his stomach.

F.H. Father died with Ca bladder. Mother died with diabetes. no sibling

By systems:

EENT: Eyesight not as good as it used to be. Has some ringing in the ears. No difficulty swallowing. Funduscopic normal. no hemorrhages. no edema.

CVR: No cough or sob. Heart ok. Occasional swelling of the feet which goes down at night.(simple salt retention will abate at night whereas edema due to heart failure or kidney failure does not abate at night. No pains in the chest.

G.I. BM regular. normal color. No pains in abd. Has heartburn relieved by tums or alka seltzer

G.U. neg

P.X. Well looking elderly man in no acute distress

EENT: normal

CVR: HR regular. No M. or thrills. 1 plus pitting edema bilaterally. Chest clear B130/75

G.I. LS and K not palp. no masses or viscera palp

Ext: 1 plus pitting edema

Rectal: Mucosa clear Prostate small and smooth.

DX: This is a rather typical story of Labryinthitis:

Discussion. One is tipped off by the paucity of findings. BP normal. No Weight loss. Condition is made worse by sudden movement of the head. On closer questioning, I found that the patient salted everything even before tasting the food. He had been using tums and alka seltzer which is laden with sodium. He had minimal edema. Had noticed some dimunition of hearing.

Treatment: Sometimes nothing helps—One should limit sodium in the diet and begin treatment by taking antivert.

Incarcerated Inguinal Hernia with Bowel Obstruction

C.C. pain in the abdomen in a 50 year old man

P.I. This all began 3 days ago when the patient noted some nausea. At the same time, he began to bloat –had no bowel movement s and occasionally passed a small amount of gas. His appetite diminished and he began to vomit (now the vomitus smells like feces—a sure sign of obstruction) He has been afebrile. His pain in the abdomen has gradually increased until it has become constant and unrelenting and now his belly is sore.

P.H.   none significant

         takes no medication

         never hospitalized

F.H. negative

By systems—neg

Physical exam

a healthy appearing 50 year old who complains of abdominal pain and bloating.

EENT   negative (there is no jaundice in the sclera—what am I thinking?)

CVR—somewhat SOB (due to the abdominal distention)

G.I.

Bloated and can feel loops of bowel—hyperresonant to percussion—no masses or viscera are palpable—somewhat distant tinkling bowel sounds and overall tenderness

G.U. small knot which is exquisitly tender in the right groin—(always undress the patient—never try to examine thru a keyhole) When questioned about a rupture, the patient stated he had had a rupture for years, but it had never bothered him!

LAB—WBC increased with a shift to the left

STAT X-ray—flat plate of abdomen revealed distended loops of small bowel—suggesting small bowel obstruction

DIAGNOSIS; incarcerated inguinal hernia with bowel obstruction

Treatment—Immediate referral to a surgeon for surgical release and repair of hernia

Patent Urachus

C.C. My belly button is sore and smells (35 year old woman)

P.I. Began one week ago—now belly button is sore, weeping and crusty and has a bad odor—there is no fever

P.X. No positive findings except a crusty umbilicus which is sore to the touch

Lab: urinalysis is normal (rule out sugar)

DIAGNOSIS; Patent Urachus

This is a patent urachus which drains and becomes infected periodically. It should be treated with hot soaks (epsom salts) and an antibiotic. Then the patient should be referred to a surgeon for excision and closure of the umbilicus. This is truly a congenital condition in that the umbilical cord never does completely atrophy and seal off. –Thus the drainage which is fecal and the skin gradually burns due to the ph in the small intestine and the cellulitis develops. It is originally a chemical cellulitis which becomes secondarily infected.

www.ingramcontent.com/pod-product-compliance
Lightning Source LLC
Chambersburg PA
CBHW031302280526
45784CB00004B/1956